Student First Aid

Subject	Section	Page
Contents		01
Introduction	01	02
Course information		02
What is first aid?	02	03
The aims of first aid		03
Responsibilities		04
Consent		04
Contacting the emergency services		05
Prioritising treatment		06
Infection control		06
Primary survey	03	07
Check for dangers		07
Check for a response		07
Opening the airway		08
Checking for breathing		08
CPR for a non-breathing casualty		09
Recovery position	04	10
Casualty assessment		10
Recovery position		11
Resuscitation and AED	05	14
Principles of resuscitation		14
Resuscitation procedure		15
Chain of survival		18
Defibrillation using an AED		19
Adult basic life support diagram		25

Subject	Section	Page
Choking	06	26
Choking – responsive casualty		27
Choking – unresponsive casualty		29
Common injuries	07	30
Concussion		30
Skull fracture		32
Types of wounds		34
Types of bleeding		34
Treatment of bleeding		35
Nosebleeds		36
Minor cuts and grazes		37
Bruising		39
Minor burns and scalds		40
The musculoskeletal system		42
Closed fracture		43
Support sling		44
Elevated sling		46
Open fracture		47
Dislocations		48
Sprains and strains		49

GW00630708

Student First Aid is published by: **Nuco Training Ltd**

COURSE INFORMATION

Student First Aid

You must attend and successfully complete the 3-hour Student First Aid course to attain the FAA Level 2 Award in Student First Aid *(RQF)* qualification. The qualification is valid for a 3 year period from your achievement date *(subject to assessment)*.

The minimum classroom contact time of three hours can be delivered in one day or spread over a maximum period of 12-months, ensuring that each session is a minimum of one hour. 'Contact hours' refer to teaching and practical time and do not include lunch and breaks etc.

Assessment details

The qualification is assessed through practical demonstration and a multiple-choice question paper. You must successfully pass both the written and practical assessments to achieve the qualification.

Practical assessments

Scenarios will be set to enable you to demonstrate your knowledge and practical skills. During the practical assessments, you will be asked a related oral question by the Trainer/Assessor. The practical assessments are ongoing throughout the course, but the Trainer/Assessor will make you aware of when the assessments take place.

The practical assessments will include:

- **Primary survey and recovery position**
- **CPR and the safe use of an AED**
- **Choking**

Written assessment

In addition to the practical assessment, you must successfully complete a written multiple-choice question assessment paper at the end of the course.

Refresher training

It is strongly recommended that you undertake annual refresher training during your three-year certification period. Although not mandatory, this will help you maintain your basic skills and keep up-to-date with any changes to first aid protocols.

Progression

Learners who achieve this qualification may progress on to the Award in Emergency First Aid at Work, the Award in First Aid at Work or other related qualifications within first aid.

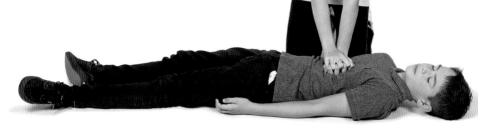

In all our lives, whether at school, work, home or at play, it is essential that we all know how to assist someone who is sick or has been injured. Your prompt, safe and effective treatment could make a difference between life and death.

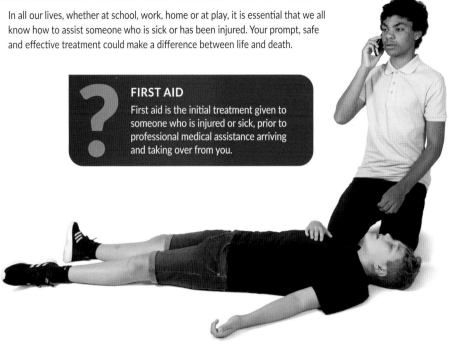

> **?**
>
> **FIRST AID**
> First aid is the initial treatment given to someone who is injured or sick, prior to professional medical assistance arriving and taking over from you.

THE AIMS OF FIRST AID

As a First Aider, your priorities for the casualty fall into the following categories:

PRESERVE life

ALLEVIATE suffering

PREVENT further illness or injury

PROMOTE recovery

For instance, if your casualty is suffering major blood loss as a result of a serious cut, then you can preserve life by offering treatment immediately and not waiting for professional help to sort it out for you. If you do nothing, then your casualty could bleed to death.

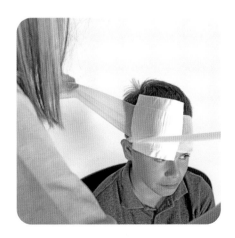

We can alleviate suffering by making the casualty more comfortable, reducing their pain levels and offering lots of care and attention.

We can prevent further illness or injury by applying a secure sterile dressing on the injured part in order to control the blood loss and prevent the risk of infection.

We can promote recovery by treating the casualty for shock and calling for an ambulance.

RESPONSIBILITIES

A First Aider has a number of responsibilities when dealing with an incident. It is very important that the incident is dealt with confidently and safely. The safety for all is important, including you, the casualty and any bystanders.

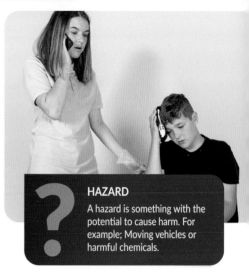

Your responsibilities can be broken up into the following categories:

- **Arriving at the scene**
- **Identifying hazards**
- **Dealing with casualties**
- **Casualty communication**
- **Contacting the emergency services**
- **Prioritising the first aid treatment**
- **Clearing up process and infection control**

? HAZARD
A hazard is something with the potential to cause harm. For example; Moving vehicles or harmful chemicals.

CONSENT

A responsive adult must agree to receive first aid treatment. Expressed consent means that the casualty gives their permission to receive care and treatment. To obtain consent, first identify yourself, tell them about your level of training and ask if it's ok to help them.

Implied consent means that permission to perform first aid care on an unresponsive casualty is assumed. This is based on the idea that a reasonable person would give their permission to receive lifesaving treatment if they were able to.

When caring for vulnerable groups such as children and the elderly, then consent must be gained from a parent, family member or legal guardian. When life-threatening situations exist and the parent, family member or legal guardian is not available, you must provide first aid care based on implied consent.

Common sense

It is necessary to apply common sense. Never attempt skills that exceed your training. Always ask a responsive casualty for permission before giving care. Call for an ambulance immediately if no first aid treatment is given.

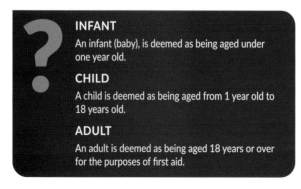

? INFANT
An infant (baby), is deemed as being aged under one year old.

CHILD
A child is deemed as being aged from 1 year old to 18 years old.

ADULT
An adult is deemed as being aged 18 years or over for the purposes of first aid.

CONTACTING THE EMERGENCY SERVICES

As soon as you have identified the extent of the injury or illness, then it may be necessary to contact the emergency services.

The emergency services can be contacted by dialling 999 or 112.

They will require vital information about the condition of the casualty so that the call can be prioritised. Activate the speaker function on the phone to aid communication with the ambulance service.

They will also require specific details about the location of the incident. It is important to have the full details of where you are, particularly if the premises are large and have multi-floors or other buildings to consider. Your bystander could manage this for you by meeting the emergency services and guiding them to the incident.

Remember **LIONEL** when making this call:

L Location

I Incident

O Other services

N Number of casualties

E Extent of injuries

L Location - repeat

?

DIAL 999

Only dial 999 if it is necessary and consider other services such as Police and Fire, dependent on the incident.

PRIORITISING YOUR FIRST AID TREATMENT

Breathing – deal with casualties who are not breathing normally first

Bleeding – deal with any major bleeding and treat the casualty for shock

Burns/breaks – treat burns and immobilise any bone injuries

Other conditions – treat appropriately

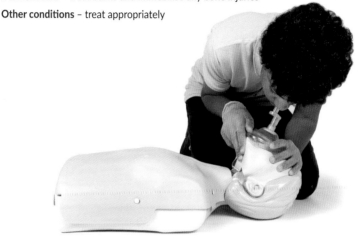

THE CLEARING UP PROCESS AND INFECTION CONTROL

You must minimise the risk of infection from the beginning when dealing with any first aid incident. This applies to you, the casualty and any bystanders. Similarly, when the casualty has been treated it is vital that any used materials are disposed of correctly.

- Wash your hands and wear disposable gloves
- Avoid coughing and sneezing over the wound and avoid touching it
- Dispose of all used materials *(including gloves)* in an appropriately marked *(orange/yellow)* plastic bag
- Dispose of sharp items, including syringes and needles, in a purpose-made sharps bin and dispose of it appropriately. It may mean taking it to your local hospital for correct disposal

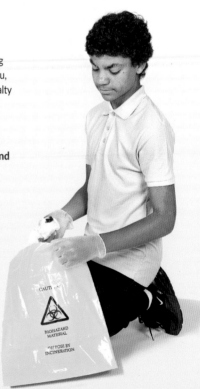

The primary survey is a quick way to find out if your casualty has any life-threatening conditions in order of priority. It's also used to make sure the area is safe before you offer to help them.

The contents of the primary survey can be remembered easily by using the memory aid **DR ABC**.

DANGERS

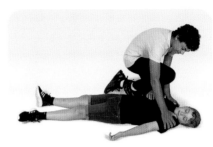

The area must be safe before you offer your casualty any treatment. Safe for you primarily, not forgetting any bystanders and of course your casualty. Failing to do this could result in you having more casualties to deal with, which could include yourself!

RESPONSE

Approach the casualty, ideally from their feet. This reduces the risk of the casualty hyper-extending their neck should they be responsive.

YOU CAN PERFORM A RESPONSIVE CHECK BY USING THE AVPU SCALE

Alert	If they are fully responsive, then ascertain the extent of their injury and deal with it appropriately.
Voice	**"Are you all right?"** If they are not alert, then see if they will respond to a voice command.
Place	**your hands on their shoulders and gently shake them.** If they don't respond to a voice command, then try shaking them gently by the shoulders. NB: do not shake them if you suspect a spinal or head injury.
Unresponsive	If there is no response at all, they must be deemed as being unresponsive.

If your casualty responds, leave them in the position in which you find them providing there is no further danger. Try to find out what is wrong with them and treat accordingly.

Call for professional medical help if it is needed and reassess them regularly.

If you are on your own, you should shout for help. Ideally, you should never leave your casualty on their own.

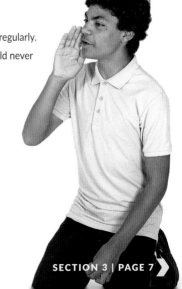

A bystander can be a great benefit to you such as:

- **Calling for an ambulance**
- **Managing crowds and hazards**
- **Fetching the First Aid kit and defibrillator if you have one**
- **Consoling relatives and friends**
- **Helping you if they are trained to do so**
- **Cleaning up**
- **A support for you**

A AIRWAY

Turn the casualty onto their back and then open the airway using the head tilt and chin lift method:

- **Place your hand on their forehead and gently tilt their head back**
- **With two fingertips under the point of their chin, lift the chin to open the airway**
- **Be careful not to press on the fleshy part under the chin as it could restrict the airway**

Support their head in this position in order to perform a breathing check.

B BREATHING

Look, listen and feel for normal breathing for no more than 10 seconds.

Look	for chest movement
Listen	at their mouth for breath sounds
Feel	for air on your cheek

In the first few minutes after cardiac arrest, a casualty may be barely breathing or taking infrequent, noisy gasps. This is often termed agonal breathing or gasping and must **not** be confused with normal breathing.

If you have any doubt whether breathing is normal, act as if it is **not** normal and prepare to commence CPR.

The casualty who is **unresponsive** and **not breathing normally** is in cardiac arrest and requires CPR. Immediately following cardiac arrest, blood flow to the brain is reduced to virtually zero, which may cause seizure-like episodes that may be confused with epilepsy. You should be suspicious of cardiac arrest with any casualty that presents seizure-like symptoms and carefully assess whether they are breathing normally.

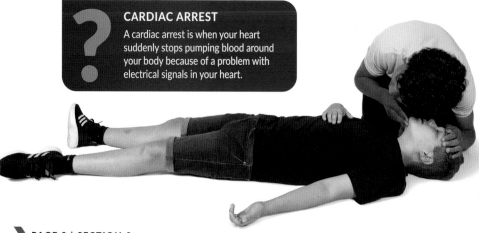

? CARDIAC ARREST

A cardiac arrest is when your heart suddenly stops pumping blood around your body because of a problem with electrical signals in your heart.

CPR FOR A NON-BREATHING CASUALTY

If your casualty is **not breathing normally**, then you must call for an ambulance immediately. If you have a bystander at hand, then send them to make this important call so that you can commence cardiopulmonary resuscitation *(CPR)* without delay.

Stay with the casualty when making this call if possible. If you are able to, activate the speaker function on your phone to aid communication between you and the emergency services.

If your casualty is breathing normally and has no major physical trauma, they should be placed in the recovery position and an ambulance should be summoned.

If your casualty has sustained physical trauma, then the injuries should be treated accordingly and the casualty left in the position found.

However, if you believe their airway is at risk, then the recovery position should be used.

Ensure that you monitor the casualty's breathing whilst waiting for the ambulance.

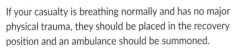

? CPR

CPR stands for cardiopulmonary resuscitation. It is an emergency procedure which is attempted to return life to a person who is in cardiac arrest (not breathing normally for themselves). CPR combines chest compressions with rescue breaths to help transport oxygen around the body. (covered in module 5)

Once you have completed your primary survey and established that your casualty is breathing normally, you will need to assess the casualty's injuries and condition, regardless of whether they are responsive or not.

CASUALTY ASSESSMENT

In order to make a diagnosis of their condition, there are three key factors to consider. By making this diagnosis correctly, it should determine the treatment you offer them. In all cases, your priority is to maintain an open airway and to ensure that they are breathing normally.

History

- Ask your casualty or bystanders what happened
- Examine the environment for obvious signs relating to the incident
- Ask your casualty about their condition. Do they have their own medication? Has it happened before? Where does it hurt? How painful is it?
- Ask the casualty their name. Is there any family present that could answer the questions about their condition?

Signs

- What can you see in respect of the injury or condition?
- Use all your other senses. What can you smell, hear and feel?

Symptoms

This is how the casualty will be feeling. Ask them how they are feeling.

- Communication is very important to ascertain the extent of their injury/illness
- Continue to question their wellbeing throughout your assessment as they may have deteriorated which may influence your decision on the appropriate treatment

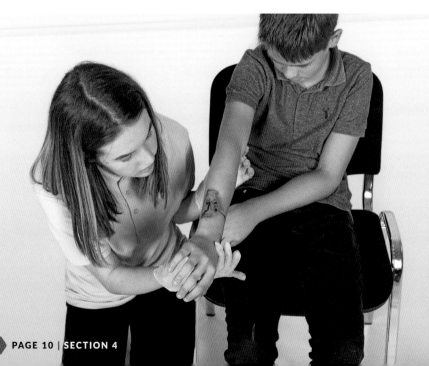

THE RECOVERY POSITION

If your casualty is unresponsive, but breathing normally, with no evidence of major physical trauma, then your priority is to ensure that their airway is not compromised in any way and that it remains open. Rather than leaving them on their back or in a slumped position, then an effective way of achieving this is to place them in the recovery position.

Whilst the casualty remains in this position, it will allow vomit to drain from the mouth and prevent them from rolling onto their back should you have to leave them.

1 Remove the casualty's glasses, if present

2 Kneel beside the casualty and make sure that both their legs are straight

3 Place the arm nearest to you out at a right angle to their body, elbow bent with the hand palm-up. Do not force the arm, let it fall naturally, but close to this position

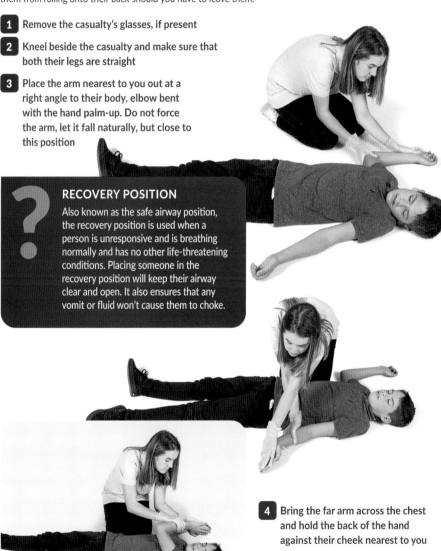

? RECOVERY POSITION

Also known as the safe airway position, the recovery position is used when a person is unresponsive and is breathing normally and has no other life-threatening conditions. Placing someone in the recovery position will keep their airway clear and open. It also ensures that any vomit or fluid won't cause them to choke.

4 Bring the far arm across the chest and hold the back of the hand against their cheek nearest to you

5 Grab hold of the far leg with your other hand and raise the knee so that their foot is kept to the floor. This will be your lever for rolling them over

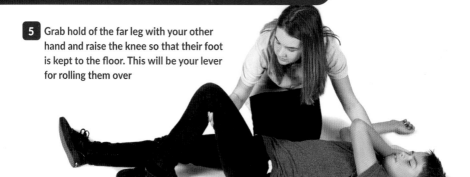

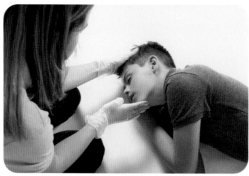

6 Keeping their hand pressed against their cheek, pull on the far leg to roll them towards you onto their side with their head supported all the way

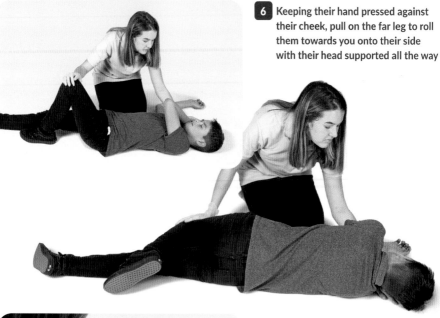

7 Tilt the head back to make sure that the airway remains open

8 If necessary, adjust the hand under their cheek to keep the head tilted and facing downwards to allow liquid material to drain from the mouth

9 Adjust the upper leg so that both the hip and knee are bent at right angles

10 Check breathing regularly

11 If you have a bystander available to you, then this is the time to send them to call for an ambulance ensuring they have all the appropriate information and in particular, the condition of the casualty

12 If you have no bystander, you must call for an ambulance yourself

Pregnant women

Always put an unresponsive pregnant woman in the recovery position on her left side. This prevents compression of the inferior vena cava (large vein) by the uterus, which could be fatal for both the mother and the child.

Suspected spinal injury

If you suspect a spinal injury and you cannot maintain an open airway in the position you found them, care must be taken in moving them. Keep the casualty's back straight and support the head throughout. It would be extremely useful to have help in moving the casualty. The trained person should assume control when moving them.

If they have to be kept in the recovery position for more than 30 minutes, turn them to the opposite side to relieve the pressure on the lower arm. You must continue to monitor their breathing whilst waiting for the emergency services to take over. If they stop breathing normally, then you must call the emergency services with an update and commence CPR immediately.

It will also be worth monitoring and noting other changes such as colouration of the skin, their temperature and responsiveness levels.

CARDIOPULMONARY RESUSCITATION (CPR)

Cardiopulmonary resuscitation *(CPR)* is an emergency procedure which is attempted in an effort to return life to a person who is not breathing normally for themselves.

This procedure combines chest compressions with rescue breaths. The chest compression replaces the heart's ability to pump oxygenated blood around the body, particularly to the vital organs such as the brain.

Rescue breathing provides the casualty, who is unable to breathe normally for themselves, valuable oxygen that is transported around the body by the chest compressions.

Without oxygen, brain damage can occur within three minutes. Therefore, your immediate action is paramount.

Referring back to the primary survey, i.e. DR ABC, then you will have established that your casualty is not breathing normally.

Your immediate action now is to contact the emergency services and ask for an ambulance ensuring that you state that your casualty is not breathing normally.

If you have a bystander at hand, then send them to make this important call. You can also ask your bystander to find and bring an Automated External Defibrillator *(AED)* if one is available.

If you are able to, activate the speaker function on your phone to aid communication between you and the emergency services.

Start CPR without delay.

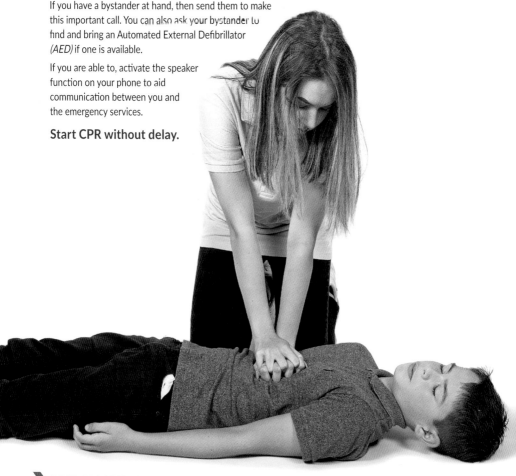

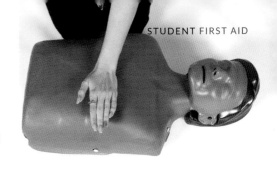

1 START WITH CHEST COMPRESSIONS

- Kneel by the side of your casualty
- Place the heel of one hand in the centre of the casualty's chest *(which is the lower half of the casualty's breastbone (sternum)*

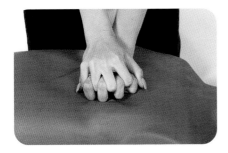

- Place the heel of your other hand on top of the first hand
- Interlock the fingers of your hands and ensure that pressure is not applied over their ribs. Do not apply any pressure over the upper abdomen or the bottom end of the sternum
- Position yourself vertically above their chest and, with your arms straight, press down on the sternum approximately 5cm *(but not more than 6cm)*

- After each compression, release all the pressure on the chest without losing contact between your hands and the sternum *(do not lean on the chest)*
- Repeat 30 chest compressions at a speed of 100 – 120 compressions per minute with as few interruptions as possible
- Compression and release should take an equal amount of time

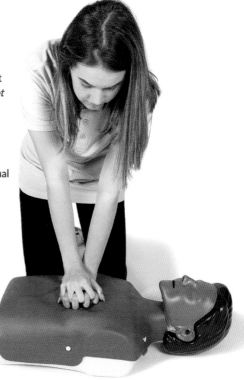

2 GIVE 2 RESCUE BREATHS

After 30 chest compressions open the airway using the head tilt and chin lift method.

- Pinch the soft part of their nose closed using the index finger and thumb of your hand on their forehead

- Allow their mouth to open, but maintain chin lift

- Take a normal breath and place your lips around their mouth, making sure that you have a good seal

- Blow steadily into their mouth whilst watching for their chest to rise, taking about one second as in normal breathing; this is an effective rescue breath

- Maintaining head tilt and chin lift, watch for their chest to fall as air comes out

- Take another normal breath and blow into the casualty's mouth once more to achieve a total of two effective rescue breaths. Do not interrupt compressions by more than 10 seconds to deliver two breaths. Then return your hands without delay to the correct position on the sternum and give a further 30 chest compressions

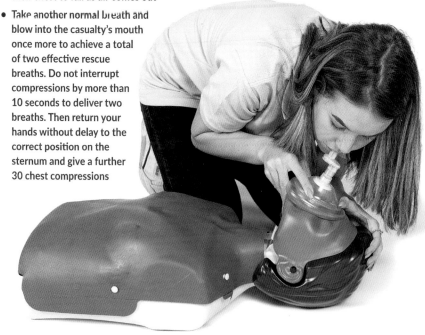

If the initial rescue breath of each sequence does not make the chest rise as in normal breathing, then, before your next attempt:

- Check the casualty's mouth and remove any visible obstruction

- Re-check that there is adequate head tilt and chin lift

- Do not attempt more than two breaths each time before returning to chest compressions

In order to reduce the risk of cross-contamination, there are various protective shields and masks available that will significantly reduce this risk.

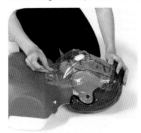 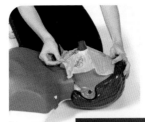 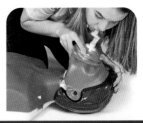

Repeat 30 compressions and 2 breaths until;

- A health professional tells you to stop
- The casualty is definitely waking up, moving, opening their eyes and breathing normally
- You become exhausted

? CROSS-CONTAMINATION
The process by which bacteria or germs are unintentionally transferred from one person to another, possibly with harmful effects.

It is rare for CPR alone to restart the heart. Unless you are certain the casualty has recovered, continue with CPR.

Signs the casualty has recovered include:

- Waking up
- Moving
- Opens eyes

AND

- They start breathing normally again

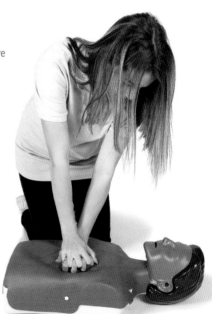

Be prepared to restart CPR immediately if the casualty worsens.

It must be emphasised that if you are unable to give rescue breaths for whatever reason, then you must continue with chest-compression-only CPR.

If there is more than one rescuer present, another should take over CPR every 1-2 minutes to avoid fatigue. Ensure the minimum delay during the changeover of rescuers and do not interrupt chest compressions.

IF YOU HAVE ACCESS TO AN AED

As soon as it arrives, switch it on and attach the electrode pads on the casualty's chest. Follow the voice prompts. If more than one rescuer is present, CPR should be continued whilst the electrode pads are being attached to the chest.

THE CHAIN OF SURVIVAL

It is critical that you follow this chain when you are dealing with a casualty who is not breathing normally.

- **Early recognition and call for help**

  Recognise those at risk of cardiac arrest and call for help in the hope that early treatment can prevent arrest.

- **Early CPR**

  Start CPR to buy time until medical help arrives.

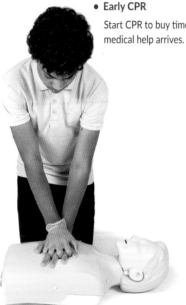

- **Early defibrillation**

  Defibrillators give an electric shock to re-organise the rhythm of the heart. Defibrillation within 3–5 minutes of cardiac arrest can produce survival rates as high as 50–70%. Each minute of delay to defibrillation reduces the probability of survival by 10%.

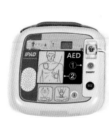
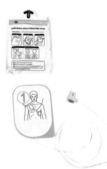

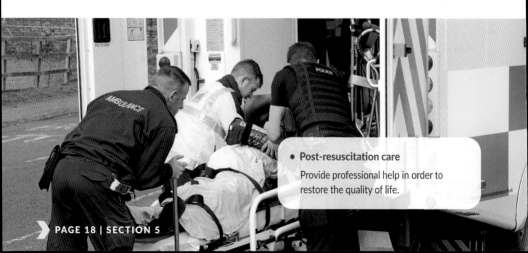

- **Post-resuscitation care**

  Provide professional help in order to restore the quality of life.

DEFIBRILLATION USING AN AED

When the AED arrives you must immediately unpack it and prepare to fix the pads to the casualty. If you have trained help, then allow them to continue with CPR until you are ready. If not, then stop CPR and unpack it yourself.

If your casualty is wearing a wired bra, then this must be removed or cut through to expose the chest, particularly the area where the pads are to be fixed. Similarly, if your casualty is wearing jewellery that may come into contact with the pads, then it must be removed.

The majority of pads will be clearly marked on where they should be fixed. Depending on the make and model of the AED, the pads will generally come as two separate pads. Some will come as a single pad. Ensure that the film that is protecting the sticky pads is removed.

If your casualty has a pacemaker fitted, then ensure that the pads are placed at least 10cms away from it.

Do not place the pads directly on top of it. A pacemaker should be clearly identifiable, from a scar or what appears to be a small plate under the skin.

?

AED

AED stands for automated external defibrillator. It is a lightweight, electronic, portable device that delivers an electric shock through the chest wall to the heart. The shock can potentially stop an irregular heart beat and allow a normal rhythm to resume following cardiac arrest.

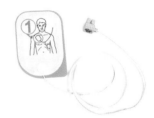

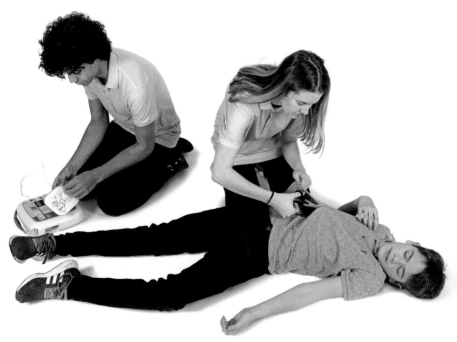

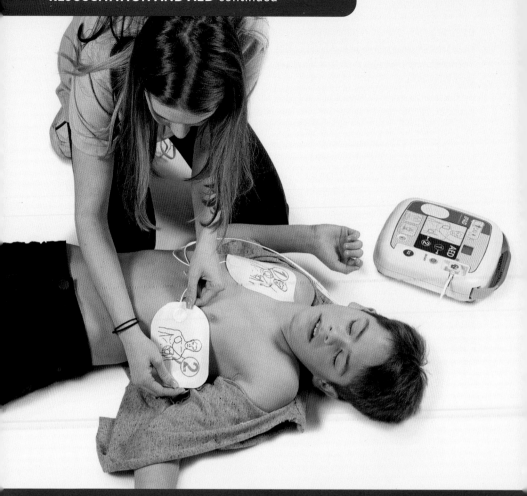

Most AED pads are labelled left and right or carry a picture of the placement. It does not matter if these pads are reversed. What is important is that should they be placed the wrong way round, they must be left in place because the adhesive may well be removed or compromised if you swap them around.

In respect of switching the AED on, they will vary from one AED to another. Some will switch themselves on as soon as the lid is removed or opened. Others will have a button to press to switch it on.

It is important that you familiarise yourself with the AED you have.

All AED's will have a voice prompt and it is important that you follow these prompts.

Some AED's will also have a screen giving you the commands. This can be a very useful aid for those who are hard of hearing.

It is important from here on in to follow these prompts as soon as the pads are connected and the AED is switched on.

The AED will need to analyse the heart's rhythm. You will be prompted to ensure that no-one is touching the casualty, including yourself. Anyone touching the casualty could have an adverse effect on detecting the correct rhythm of your casualty's heart.

Dependent on the model you have, the analysis will automatically happen or you may have to push the 'Analyse' button.

You have to take control of the situation and move people away from the casualty.

Your next prompt could be to shock the casualty. Your AED may do this automatically or you may have to press the 'Shock' button.

Again, manage the situation and ensure that no-one is touching the casualty.

Keep following the prompts from the AED.

If you are prompted to commence CPR, then quality CPR is important. Ensure that you compress at the right depth *(5-6cms)* and at the right speed *(100-120 chest compressions per minute)*.

In essence, you must continue with CPR until the AED tells you to stop to either analyse the casualty's heart rhythm or it decides that a shock should be given.

Under the current resuscitation guidelines, you will be administering CPR for two minutes before the AED will prompt you to stop in order for it to analyse the heart's rhythm.

You must continue to follow the prompts until professional medical help takes over from you, your casualty recovers or you become too exhausted to continue.

Recovery will mean that your casualty shows signs of regaining responsiveness, such as coughing, opening their eyes, speaking or moving purposefully AND they start to breathe normally for themselves. To ensure they are breathing normally, conduct a breathing check.

If you are confident that they are breathing normally, place them in the recovery position with the pads attached and connected to the AED.

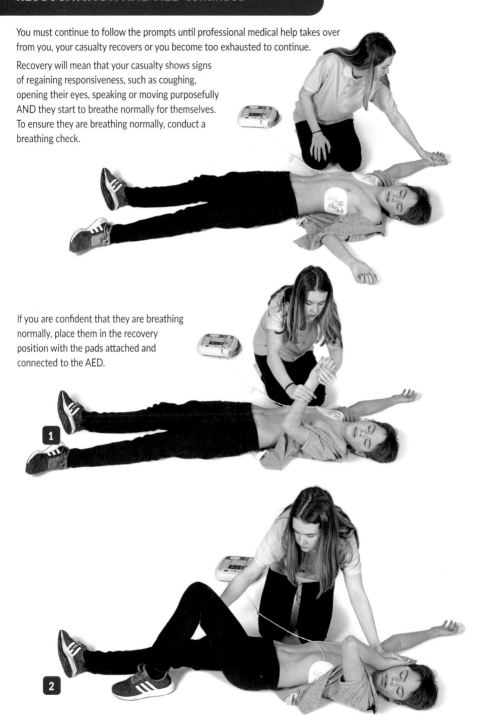

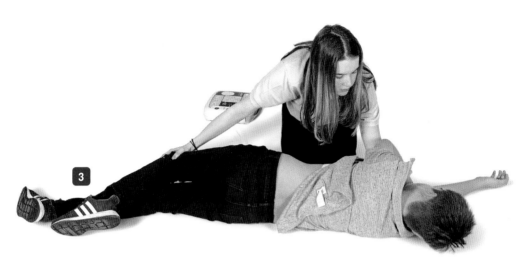

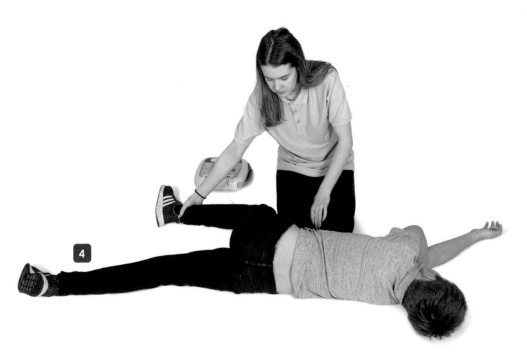

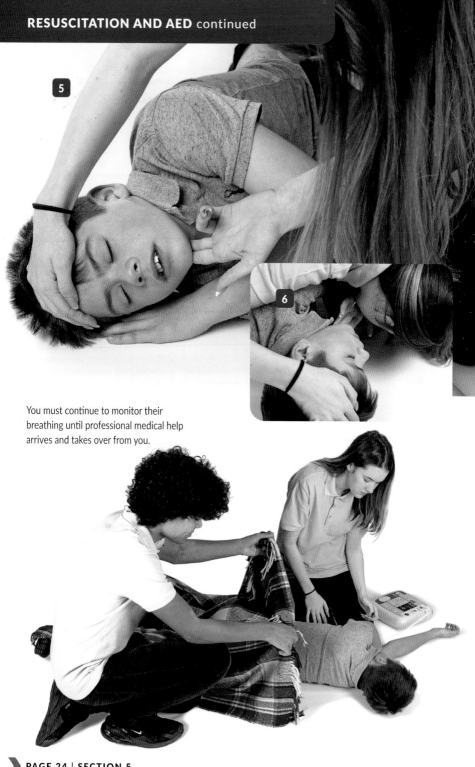

5

6

You must continue to monitor their breathing until professional medical help arrives and takes over from you.

ADULT BASIC LIFE SUPPORT

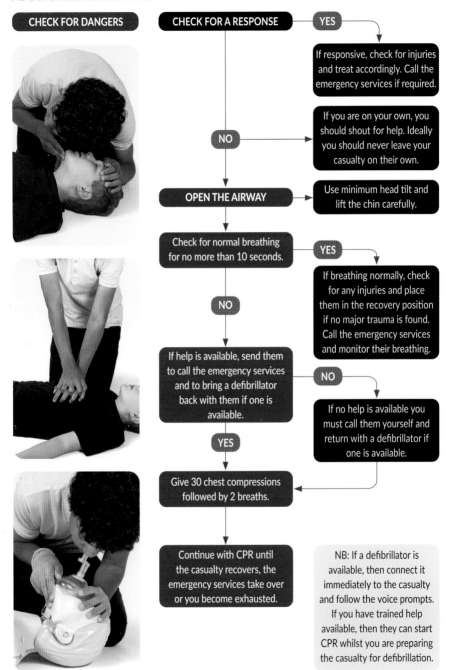

CHECK FOR DANGERS

CHECK FOR A RESPONSE — **YES**

If responsive, check for injuries and treat accordingly. Call the emergency services if required.

NO

If you are on your own, you should shout for help. Ideally you should never leave your casualty on their own.

OPEN THE AIRWAY

Use minimum head tilt and lift the chin carefully.

Check for normal breathing for no more than 10 seconds. — **YES**

NO

If breathing normally, check for any injuries and place them in the recovery position if no major trauma is found. Call the emergency services and monitor their breathing.

If help is available, send them to call the emergency services and to bring a defibrillator back with them if one is available. — **NO**

If no help is available you must call them yourself and return with a defibrillator if one is available.

YES

Give 30 chest compressions followed by 2 breaths.

Continue with CPR until the casualty recovers, the emergency services take over or you become exhausted.

NB: If a defibrillator is available, then connect it immediately to the casualty and follow the voice prompts. If you have trained help available, then they can start CPR whilst you are preparing the casualty for defibrillation.

CHOKING

There are many factors that can contribute to a respiratory disorder including asthma, hypoxia *(lack of oxygen)*, smoke inhalation and choking.

Choking is probably the most common of the disorders and probably the most distressing to suffer and to deal with.

Your immediate treatment is required.

RECOGNITION OF SOMEONE CHOKING

- Difficulty in speaking and breathing
- Coughing or gagging
- Clutching at the throat and pointing to the mouth
- Pale, grey/blue skin tone in the later stages *(cyanosis)*
- Ultimately – unresponsiveness

If your casualty shows signs of a mild or partial airway obstruction then:

- Encourage them to continue coughing, but do nothing else at this stage
- Stay calm and offer plenty of encouragement and reassurance

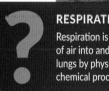

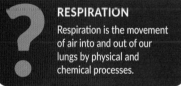

RESPIRATION

Respiration is the movement of air into and out of our lungs by physical and chemical processes.

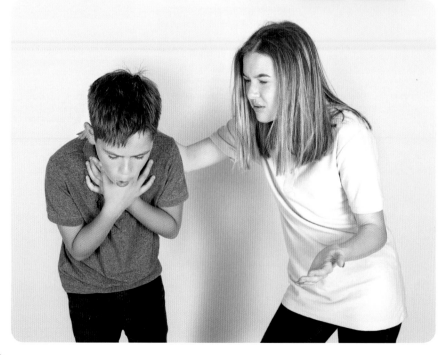

TREATMENT FOR A SEVERE AIRWAY OBSTRUCTION FOR AN ADULT

- Check their mouth and remove any obvious obstruction

Bend them forward and give up to five back blows

- Stand to the side and slightly behind your casualty
- Support the chest with one hand and lean them forward so that when the obstructing object is dislodged it comes out of the mouth rather than to go further down the airway
- Give up to five sharp blows between their shoulder blades with the heel of your other hand

Check to see if each back blow has relieved the airway obstruction.
The aim is to relieve the obstruction with each blow rather than to give all five unnecessarily.

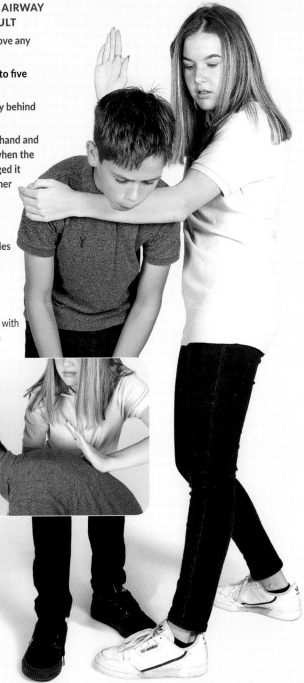

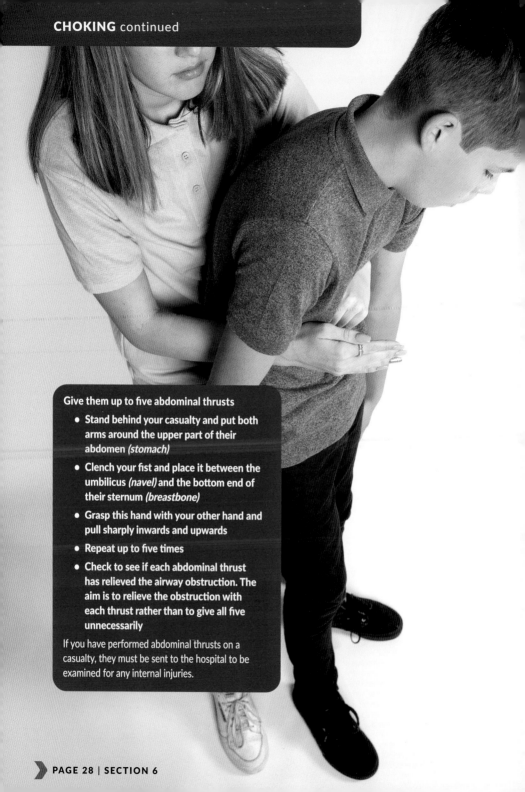

Give them up to five abdominal thrusts

- Stand behind your casualty and put both arms around the upper part of their abdomen *(stomach)*
- Clench your fist and place it between the umbilicus *(navel)* and the bottom end of their sternum *(breastbone)*
- Grasp this hand with your other hand and pull sharply inwards and upwards
- Repeat up to five times
- Check to see if each abdominal thrust has relieved the airway obstruction. The aim is to relieve the obstruction with each thrust rather than to give all five unnecessarily

If you have performed abdominal thrusts on a casualty, they must be sent to the hospital to be examined for any internal injuries.

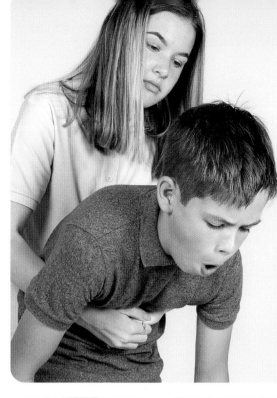

If the obstruction cannot be removed after the first cycle of back blows and abdominal thrusts, then you must call for an ambulance immediately. Repeat the process of up to five back blows followed by up to five abdominal thrusts until the casualty recovers or the emergency medical services take over from you.

TREATMENT FOR AN UNRESPONSIVE CHOKING CASUALTY

If your casualty becomes unresponsive, then help them to the floor onto their back, call 999/112 and commence CPR immediately.

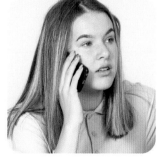

Before each rescue breath attempt, check in the mouth for any visible obstruction that can be removed easily without having to sweep the mouth with your fingers.

HEAD INJURIES

All injuries to the head are potentially dangerous and they all require a medical assessment.

You should be monitoring and looking at the following:

- Eyes
- Speech
- Movement
- Breathing
- Responsiveness

CONCUSSION

A concussion is a traumatic brain injury that may result in a bad headache, altered levels of alertness or unresponsiveness. It temporarily interferes with the way your brain works and it can affect memory, judgment, reflexes, speech, balance, coordination and sleep patterns.

Signs and symptoms

The most common signs and symptoms of concussion are:

- Evidence of a head injury *(blood or bruising)*
- Headache and nausea *(feeling sick)*
- Dizziness and loss of balance
- Confusion, such as being unaware of your surroundings
- Feeling stunned or dazed
- Disturbances with vision, such as double vision or seeing "stars" or flashing lights
- Difficulties with memory

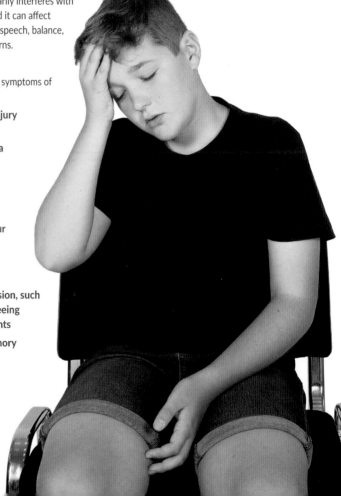

Treatment

- If they are responsive, rest them by sitting them down or lying them down with their head raised and hold a cold compress against the injury

- Keep them warm and keep talking to them

- Ensure the cold compress stays on the injury for no longer than 20 minutes

- Monitor their airway, breathing and response levels

- If they are unresponsive, you must call for an ambulance and support them in the position found

- You must recommend that they seek medical advice, particularly if they develop a headache, feel sick or they sleep more than they would normally do

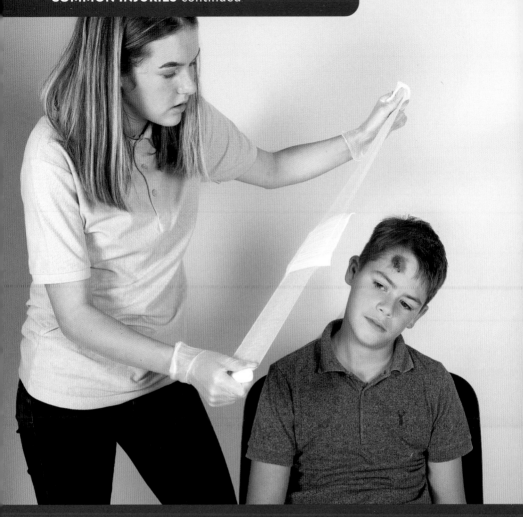

SKULL FRACTURE

A skull fracture is caused by any impact or blow to the head that is strong enough to break the cranial bones (the skull).

Specific causes can include a fall from height, a serious sports injury or a road traffic accident.

Signs and symptoms

- Evidence of trauma to the head
- Possible depression of the skull
- Bruising around the head
- Clear fluid or watery blood coming from the nose or ear
- Bloodshot eyes
- Deterioration of response levels

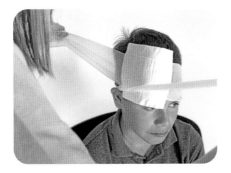
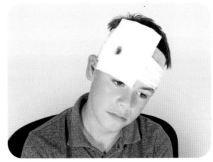

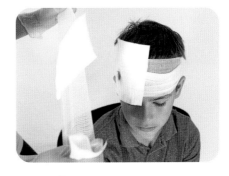

Treatment

- If you suspect a spinal injury, do not move them
- Lay them down, head and shoulders raised if you are able to move them, injured side down
- Call for an ambulance
- Monitor their airway, breathing and response levels
- Cover their ear with a sterile dressing if there is fluid running out of it
- Control the bleeding and fluid loss
- All head injuries must be advised to go to the hospital

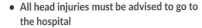

TYPES OF WOUNDS

A wound can be best described as a type of injury in which the skin is torn, cut or punctured *(an open wound)*, or where a blunt force created a contusion *(a bruise)*.

In first aid there are 6 types of wounds that you should be familiar with:

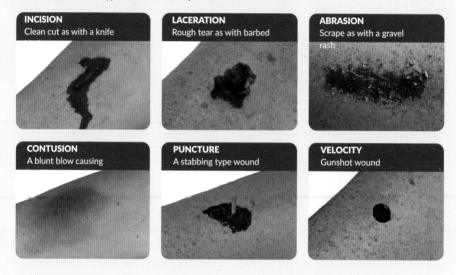

INCISION
Clean cut as with a knife

LACERATION
Rough tear as with barbed

ABRASION
Scrape as with a gravel rash

CONTUSION
A blunt blow causing

PUNCTURE
A stabbing type wound

VELOCITY
Gunshot wound

When a blood vessel is torn or severed, blood loss and shock cause the blood pressure to fall and the injured vessels will contract at the site of injury. Platelets and proteins come into contact with the injured site and plug the wound. This clotting process begins within ten minutes if the loss of blood is brought under control.

TYPES OF BLEEDING

Bleeding is classified by the type of blood vessel that is damaged.

Arterial   Pumps from the wound with the heartbeat

Venous   Gushes from the wound or pools at the site

Capillary   Oozing at the site of injury

Once you have completed your initial casualty assessment for prioritising your treatment, you must follow the guidelines for personal protection and hygiene control before you begin to treat the casualty for bleeding.

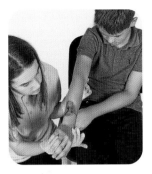 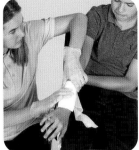 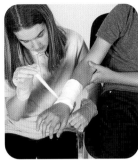

TREATMENT OF BLEEDING

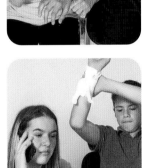

- Put on disposable gloves
- Expose and examine the wound
- Apply direct pressure with your fingers or palm, preferably over a sterile dressing or non-fluffy clean pad *(you can ask your casualty to apply this pressure)*
- Elevate and support the injured part
- Help the casualty to lie down and raise the legs if you suspect shock
- Secure the dressing with a bandage large enough to cover the wound
- If blood seeps through this dressing, remove both the dressing and bandage and apply pressure to the bleed with a new dressing
- Secure the new dressing with a bandage once the bleeding is under control
- If there is something embedded in the wound, control the bleeding by applying direct pressure on either side of the object
- Build up padding on either side of the object *(using rolled dressings)* until it is high enough for you to bandage over the top and secure the dressing
- Support the injured limb with a sling or bandaging, providing the casualty allows you to do so
- Monitor their response levels and call for an ambulance

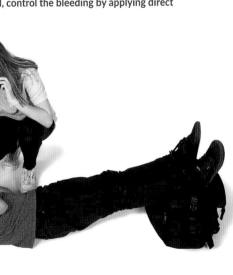

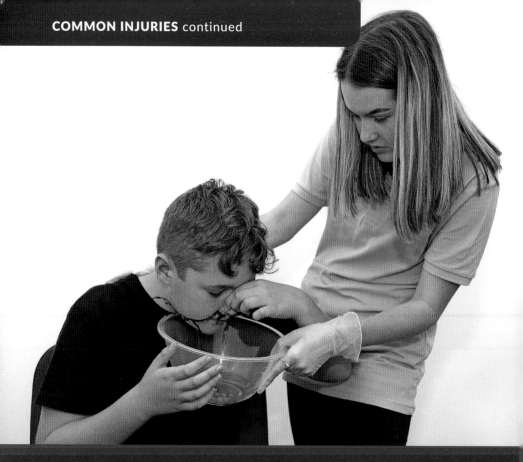

NOSEBLEEDS

A common injury that is caused generally by a direct blow or sneezing. However, high blood pressure can also cause a sudden bleed with little warning.

If the blood is watery, then it could suggest a head injury, therefore making the incident far more serious i.e. possible skull fracture.

Treatment

- Sit the casualty down and lean them forward
- Ask them to pinch the soft part of the nose as they lean forward
- Apply this pressure for 10 minutes and then release slowly
- Ask them to avoid rubbing or blowing their nose
- If you are unable to stop the bleeding, ask them to repeat the pinching process for a further 10 minutes
- If the bleeding continues beyond 30 minutes then you will need to seek medical advice
- If you suspect a head injury, then an ambulance must be summoned

If the casualty is feeling faint or sick, you may consider sitting the casualty on the floor with their back supported. This could potentially prevent a fall.

MINOR CUTS AND GRAZES

Cuts and grazes are some of the most common injuries. Minor cuts and grazes *(where only the surface layer of skin is cut or scraped off)* may bleed and feel slightly painful, but the affected area will normally scab over and heal quickly.

However, if the cut is in an area that is constantly moving, such as your knee joint, it may take longer to heal. Depending on how deep the cut is and where it is on your body, a scar may remain once the cut has healed.

Deeper cuts may damage important structures below the skin such as nerves, blood vessels or tendons. However, grazes that remove the deeper layers of skin are rare.

Most cuts and grazes can be easily treated by cleaning them thoroughly and covering them with a plaster or dressing. Please bear in mind that hypoallergenic plasters are available should your casualty have an allergy to ordinary plasters.

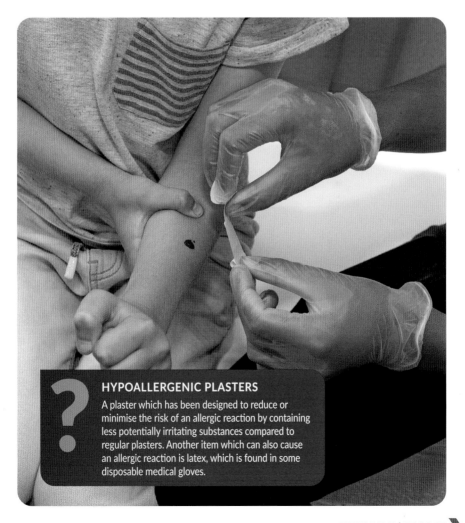

? HYPOALLERGENIC PLASTERS

A plaster which has been designed to reduce or minimise the risk of an allergic reaction by containing less potentially irritating substances compared to regular plasters. Another item which can also cause an allergic reaction is latex, which is found in some disposable medical gloves.

SEEK MEDICAL HELP IF ANY OF THE BELOW APPLY:

You think there is damage to deeper tissues: Signs include numbness *(indicating injury to a nerve)*, blood spurting from the wound or bleeding that does not stop after five minutes of continuous firm pressure.

The wound is at risk of becoming infected: For example, a cut has been contaminated with soil, faeces or a dirty blade, or fragments of material such as grit or glass which can be seen in the wound.

The wound has become infected: Signs include swelling of the affected area, pus coming from the wound, redness spreading from the wound and increasing pain. The wound cannot be closed with a plaster, or it starts to open up when it moves.

The wound will create an unwelcome scar: For example, if it occurs on a prominent part of the casualty's face.

TETANUS IMMUNISATION

If the wound has been contaminated by dirt or soil, then it is advisable to ask the casualty about their history of tetanus immunisation.

Advise to seek medical advice if:

- They have never been immunised
- If they are unsure about their history of injections

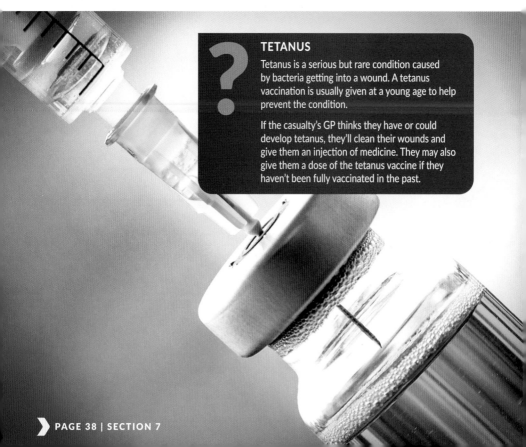

TETANUS

Tetanus is a serious but rare condition caused by bacteria getting into a wound. A tetanus vaccination is usually given at a young age to help prevent the condition.

If the casualty's GP thinks they have or could develop tetanus, they'll clean their wounds and give them an injection of medicine. They may also give them a dose of the tetanus vaccine if they haven't been fully vaccinated in the past.

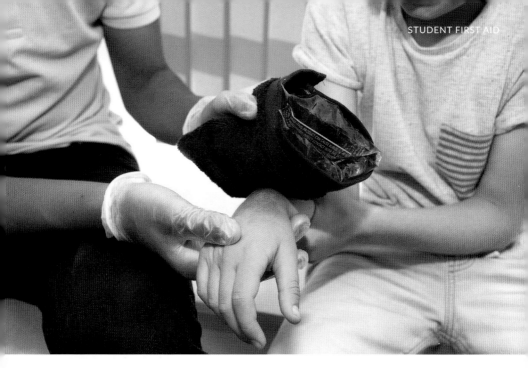

BRUISING

Bruises are bluish or purple-coloured patches that appear on the skin when tiny blood vessels *(capillaries)* break or burst underneath it. The blood from the capillaries leaks into the soft tissue under the skin causing the discolouration. Over time this fades through shades of yellow or green. Bruises often feel tender or swollen at first.

What causes bruising?

Bruising is caused by internal bleeding *(under the skin)* due to a person injuring themselves by, for example, falling over, walking into something or playing sports.

Some people are naturally more likely to bruise than others, for example, the elderly may bruise more easily because their skin is thinner and the tissue underneath is more fragile.

Treatment for bruises

Treat bruises, initially, by limiting the bleeding. You can do this by cooling the area with a cold compress *(a flannel or cloth soaked in cold water)* or an ice pack wrapped in a towel.

To make an ice pack, place ice cubes or a packet of frozen vegetables in a plastic bag and wrap them in a towel. Hold this over the affected area for at least 10 minutes.

Do not put the ice pack straight onto the skin as this will possibly cause further damage.

Most bruises will disappear after around two weeks. If the bruise is still there after two weeks, you should recommend that your casualty see their GP.

Internal bruising

Bruises don't just happen under the skin - they can also happen deeper in the body's tissues, organs and bones. While the bleeding isn't visible, the bruises can cause swelling and pain.

You should recommend that your casualty seeks medical attention or call for an ambulance if you feel the injury is of a serious nature, particularly if they have been involved in an accident.

MINOR BURNS AND SCALDS

Burns and scalds are among the most serious and painful injuries. They can be caused by a number of factors including fire, water, electricity, oils, hot surfaces, steam, chemicals and radiation.

Classification of burns

- **Superficial**

The outer layer of skin is burnt causing redness, tenderness and inflammation.

Typical factors causing this would be sunburn or touching a hot iron.

The skin is not broken or blistered.

- **Partial thickness**

The outer layer of the skin is burnt and broken causing blistering, swelling, pain and rawness.

- **Full thickness**

All the layers of skin have been damaged causing the skin to look pale, charred and waxy with fatty deposits. There may also be damage to the nerves.

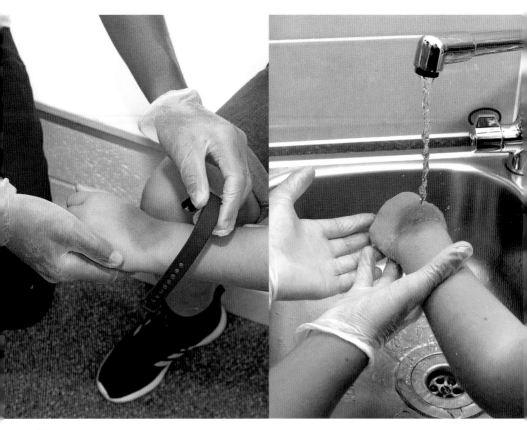

TREATMENT OF BURNS

- Ensure the area is safe, particularly from the source that created the burn or scald
- Wear disposable gloves
- If it's possible, remove the watch and any jewellery around the affected area
- Cool the burn with cool running tap water for 20 minutes
- Cover the burn with a suitable sterile dressing that is not fluffy. You can cover it with cling film if you have no appropriate dressing
- Treat the casualty for shock
- Monitor their condition throughout and call for an ambulance if it deteriorates
- Remove them to hospital if you consider it appropriate

You must not:

- Apply any form of cream, ointment or fat to the affected area
- Burst any blister that may form
- Apply any form of adhesive dressing
- Remove anything that is stuck to the affected area

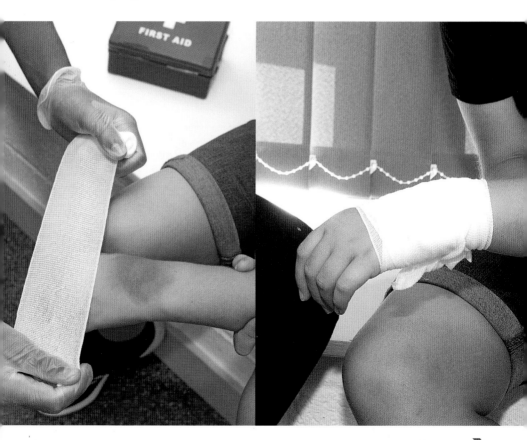

THE MUSCULOSKELETAL SYSTEM

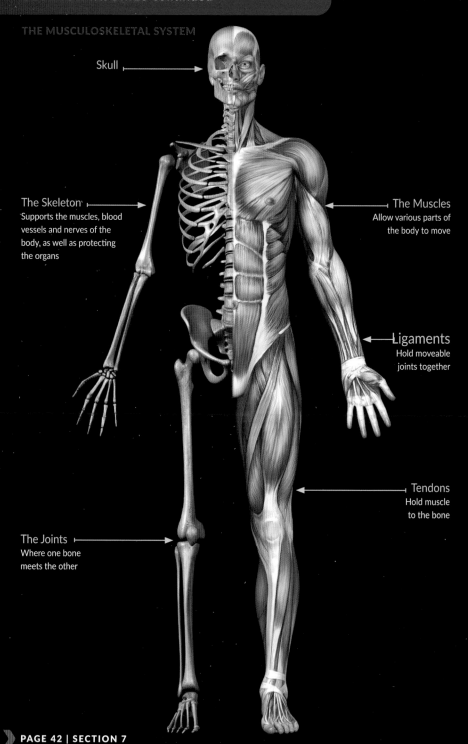

Skull

The Skeleton
Supports the muscles, blood
vessels and nerves of the
body, as well as protecting
the organs

The Muscles
Allow various parts of
the body to move

Ligaments
Hold moveable
joints together

Tendons
Hold muscle
to the bone

The Joints
Where one bone
meets the other

CLOSED FRACTURE

Signs and symptoms

- Pain
- Swelling
- Deformity
- Internal bleeding
- Bruising
- Shock

Treatment

- Immobilise the injured part to stop any movement
- Place padding around the injury for further support
- Leave the casualty in the position found unless they can move the injured part to a more comfortable position
- For additional support, particularly if there is a delay in the emergency services arriving, you could consider strapping an uninjured leg to the injured one. Use broad-fold bandages and ensure that any knots are tied to the uninjured side. Do not wrap a bandage over the fracture. If their circulation is impaired, loosen the dressings
- You MUST NOT try to realign the fracture. This should only be performed by medically trained professionals
- Do not give your casualty anything to eat or drink
- Treat for shock
- Call 999/112

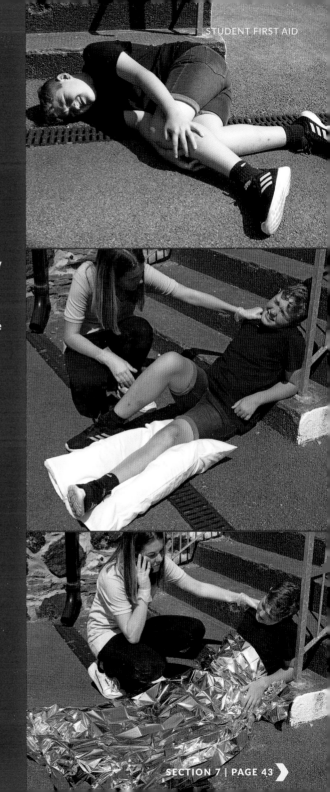

SUPPORT SLING

Injuries to the hand, wrist or arm can be very painful. This includes fractures, sprains and strains. There is little a First Aider can do other than support it and to dispatch them to hospital. In respect of support, generally speaking, the casualty will support it themselves and will not want you to move it.

If they are unable to support it themselves, then you can offer to apply a support sling using a triangular bandage.

Identify the injury to the arm and providing the arm can be bent at the elbow, offer your casualty support for it.

Pass the bandage under the injured arm with the long base running parallel with the body. The point opposite the long base should be at the elbow of the injured arm.

Bring the lower point of the bandage up over the injured arm and over the shoulder so that the two ends meet.

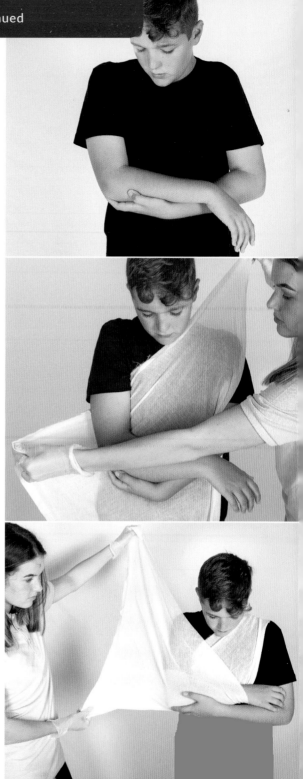

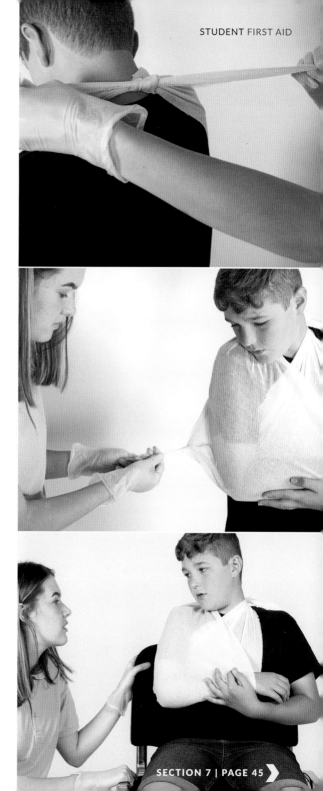

Tie off the two ends on the injured side above the collar bone. Place the two ends under the knot to act as a cushion for the knot.

Secure the trailing bandage at the elbow with a safety pin or by twisting it fairly tight and losing it by tucking it away within the sling.

Ensure that there is still circulation in the fingertips by performing a capillary refill check. Press a fingernail which should go pale. When released it should go back to normal colouration. Transport them to the hospital or call 999 if they are unable to walk.

ELEVATED SLING

An elevated sling is used for injuries affecting the shoulder, such as a dislocation.

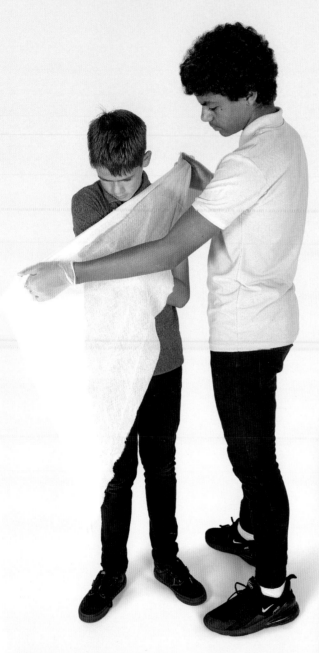

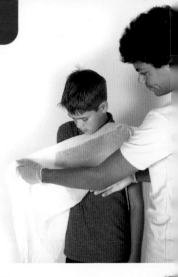

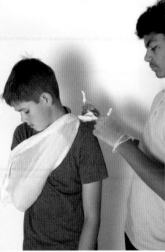

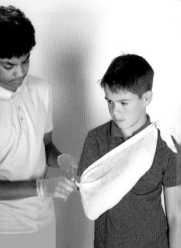

OPEN FRACTURE

Signs and symptoms

- Pain
- Deformity
- Internal bleeding
- External bleeding
- Shock

Treatment

- Call for an ambulance immediately
- Prevent any movement
- Reduce the risk of infection by wearing gloves
- Control the blood loss by dressing around the wound
- DO NOT apply any direct pressure on the protruding bone
- Use sterile non-fluffy dressings to cover the wound
- For additional support, particularly if there is a delay in the emergency services arriving, you could consider strapping an uninjured leg to the injured one
- Use broad-fold bandages and ensure that any knots are tied to the uninjured side
- Do not wrap a bandage over the fracture. If their circulation is impaired, loosen the dressings
- You MUST NOT try to realign the fracture. This should only be performed by medically trained professionals
- Treat for shock and monitor their vital signs
- Do not offer the casualty anything to eat or drink as a general anaesthetic may have to be administered when they get to the hospital

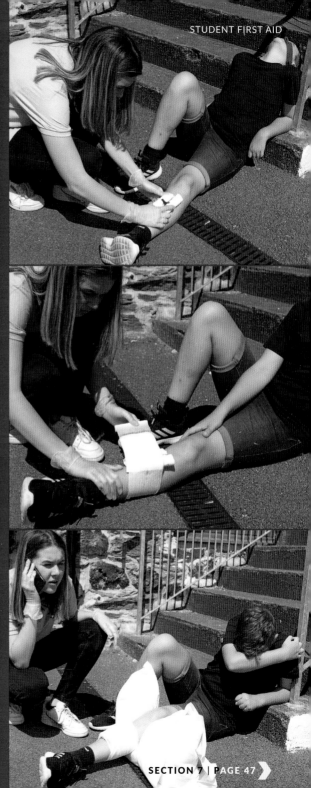

DISLOCATIONS

Dislocations are extremely painful and are often caused by a violent muscle contraction, a strong force wrenching the bone into an abnormal position or even as something as simple as turning over in bed can cause it.

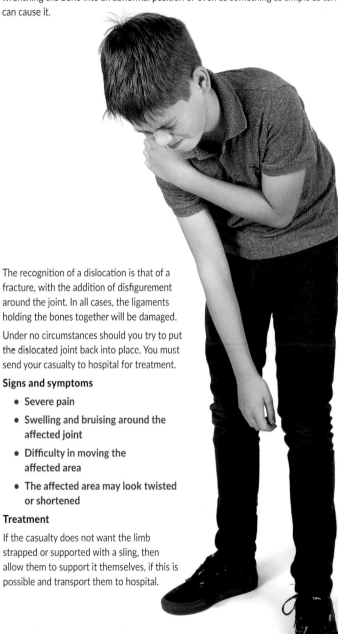

The recognition of a dislocation is that of a fracture, with the addition of disfigurement around the joint. In all cases, the ligaments holding the bones together will be damaged.

Under no circumstances should you try to put the dislocated joint back into place. You must send your casualty to hospital for treatment.

Signs and symptoms

- **Severe pain**
- **Swelling and bruising around the affected joint**
- **Difficulty in moving the affected area**
- **The affected area may look twisted or shortened**

Treatment

If the casualty does not want the limb strapped or supported with a sling, then allow them to support it themselves, if this is possible and transport them to hospital.